Critical Acclaim for James Atkinson's 'HOME WORKOUT FOR BEGINNERS'

"This is a down-to-earth, easy-to-follow guide to getting into shape. It isn't just about mere exercise; it is a workout program that goes over six weeks, and includes the motivation and lifestyle necessary to begin and carry through the program. The exercises comprise cardiovascular and resistance training, but the bonus is that you can do the exercises without bands, as well as with them. So if you don't have exercise bands, don't let that be a hindrance to beginning to get in shape and to get your mental attitude in a state to be fit. The motivational statements (that were designed as printable post signs to keep you motivated) were motivational without even beginning the program!
It's not just exercise that the book covers; it's a lifestyle – as diet and attitude are covered as well. If you are looking to improve your life through an easy-to-follow fitness program – this is the book for you."

– Ryshia Kennie

"Getting started with exercise can be really intimidating sometimes, but the author of this workout guide makes it simple and inexpensive. James Atkinson tells us that a gym membership isn't required in order to get healthy and fit, and that the long-term benefits of an everyday workout routine far outweigh the initial struggles of getting active.
Atkinson's guide is encouraging, helpful, and really easy – he describes all of the exercises outlined in the book and creates a schedule to start a healthy exercise routine. The added motivational quotes inside the guidebook are a nice touch as well, and make for a positive atmosphere.
I recommend this one for people ready to kickstart their exercise routine with an unintimidating guide."

– Avid Reader

D1364096

"This book is equipped with all I need to know about a fitness program. It talked about food consumption and types of exercises. It described how important it is to prepare physically and mentally for such a venture. And lastly, my favourite part was that it gave a workout plan with a balance so that the individual can benefit in a few new areas."

– Kay Dee

"I think, when people are brand new to exercising, it can be daunting not knowing what certain moves are; but the pictures take care of that. As usual, Jim has written a book that is straight-talking and easy to follow."

– Lucy Croft

Home
WORKOUT
for
BEGINNERS

6—Week Fitness Program
with Fat Burning Workouts &
Fitness Motivation for Weight Loss
for Life

swapfat4fit.com

Home WORKOUT *for* BEGINNERS

6—Week Fitness Program
with Fat Burning Workouts &
Fitness Motivation for Weight Loss
for Life

JAMES ATKINSON

SWAPFAT4FIT.COM
PAPERBACK EDITION

PUBLISHED BY:
JBA Publishing
http://www.swapfat4fit.com
jim@swapfat4fit.com

Book Proofing, Design & Layout by King Samuel Benson
ksb@kingsamuelbenson.com

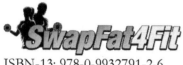

ISBN-13: 978-0-9932791-2-6

First published in 2015 / First printed in 2015
Printed in United Kingdom

TABLE OF CONTENTS

PREFACE

Hi, I'm Jim – a qualified fitness coach who is very passionate about helping people reach their potentials.

I've been a long distance runner, competing bodybuilder and served a number of years in the British army in an airborne unit (9 para sqn R.E)

You will find out a lot more about me if you visit my website:

SwapFat4Fit.com

I'd like to thank you for your purchase, and I know you will get some great weight loss and fitness results if you take on-board the information that you read.

This book will give you many of the tools you need to turn your life around and become fitter, leaner and healthier.

I have put a great focus on fitness results for the long term in these pages, and it is my opinion that this approach is the best way to go with any fitness goal.

I'll let you get stuck into the book now, but I would just like to mention that if you have any questions or comments, I would be more than happy to help you as these subjects are a passion of mine and have been for many years.

Big thanks to all of my family and friends who have been a huge influence on me. These have helped me become the positive person that I am today.

Also, a special thanks to Tammy for supporting me through everything.

INTRODUCTION

Although it is fact that you can lose weight with a strong mental attitude, a healthy diet and a few metabolism boosting tricks, I would strongly suggest that you also add a progressive exercise routine to your weight loss and "body transforming plans" as the frosting on the cake.

Having a solid progressive exercise routine will increase your fitness and weight loss results exponentially!

This book is exactly that! It is a beginner's exercise routine that can be done without the use of a gym and minimal equipment.

I have designed this routine myself using the knowledge of fitness and my own personal experiences that I have gained over the many years that I have been in this industry.

If I happened to be a beginner to fitness, overweight, recovering from an injury or unhappy with my body in any way, and I know what I know now, this is exactly what I would do to start me off!

Good luck, and please remember that I am always happy to help.

GRAB YOUR BONUS

I strongly believe that anyone can get the fitness results that they want. It just takes a bit of consistency and work.

To help you along with the diet aspect of your journey, I have created a PDF for you.

The PDF holds some of my very own recipes. Everyone who knows me knows that I love my food! But living a healthy lifestyle means that some of the best foods are out of bounds...

Or are they?

I have messed around in the kitchen and created some great recipes (and some abominations, but fortunately for you, I will not share these) that are low in fat, low in sugar and high in quality nutritional value.

As a 'thank you' for your interest in my book, I would like to offer you these 7 healthy recipes that will really help to boost your results!

Simply click this link or copy the following URL into your web browser and let me know where to send them!

http://swapfat4fit.com/reader-bonus/

Happy cooking!

CHAPTER 1

THANK YOU FOR JOINING ME

First off, I would like to thank you for your interest in my routine. I am truly appreciative of your choice and faith that you have put in my hands to get this far.

I would really like to help you to start to get into shape and remove (for good) the barriers that have been stopping you from taking those all-important first steps!

If you are reading this, there is a good chance that you have been wanting to start some kind of exercise or health kick for a while or you have simply been aware that you are getting more unfit, putting on more weight and it will just get worse as more time goes by?

The good news is that you have come to the right place! I can totally relate to this feeling and can also relate to that mountain that you feel you are about to climb.

I know how this feels, so I have designed this 6-week routine to turn that mountain into a small hill with a gentle gradient.

I have also considered cost and time. I am fully aware of today's fast-paced lifestyle, so I have tried to make this very affordable with no expensive gym memberships or expensive equipment.

This exercise plan can be done at home in a relatively short space of time and can fit into anyone's daily routine.
You will need:
- Suitable clothing and footwear (I suggest investing in):
  - ✓ A good pair of running shoes.
  - ✓ Outdoor clothing and high visibility jacket or strips for clothing.
- Exercise bands
- An exercise ball

- Focus and commitment

No excuses; there really aren't any – if you want it, you have to go and get it!

CHAPTER 2

A BIT ABOUT GENERAL FITNESS

When starting any training routine, the desired result from the training that you do is known as "The Training Effect".

This basically means that you will get the results you train for, i.e. if you train for fat loss you will actually lose fat. If you train for muscle mass, you actually gain muscle. One of the hardest phases of training is the first phase.

I know this because I have been in this situation many times. When I say first phase I mean the stage you get to after making the decision to start a training routine. At this point, you will need to get yourself into a new routine and get motivated to start training and to hit your sessions no matter what. This can be very tough, especially if you have not trained before.

It may be very hard in the first few weeks but if you persevere, you WILL get results. The compound effect basically works like this; if you have "lots of a little bit of something," you will end up with "a lot". Of course, it works both ways with the human body. If you eat a few chocolate bars every day and don't burn off the extra calories, you will put on some, or a lot of fat.

If you train consistently for a while, you will see results. Other people will notice this and start to ask questions and compliment you.

When this happens, you have reached the next phase. Now you will have seen results and want to keep them coming.

This is because you have seen the fruits of your labor and you know that what you have been working for is starting to pay off.

Year after year, gym membership numbers will go up in January, but by April have dropped back down. This is, sadly, due to people not getting past the first and, in my opinion, the hardest phase.

The number one reason people give up so fast is that they look at how far they have to go, instead of looking at how far they have gone already.

So keep going, force yourself to stick to the routine until you see these first few results – it is at this point that it will become a whole lot easier!

CHAPTER 3

HEALTH CHECK

Before you embark on any fitness routine, please consult your Doctor.

1. Do not exercise if you are unwell.
2. Stop if you feel pain, and if the pain does not subside, then see your Doctor.
3. Do not exercise if you have taken alcohol or had a large meal in the last few hours.
4. If you are taking medication, please check with your Doctor to make sure it is okay for you to exercise.
5. If in doubt at all, please check with your Doctor first – you may even want to take this routine and go through it with them. It may be helpful to ask for a blood pressure, cholesterol and weight check. You can then have these read again in a few months after exercise to see the benefit.

CHAPTER 4

FOOD

As you may be aware, food plays a very important part in creating your body composition and fueling your body. With any lifestyle change, I believe that if there are many changes going on at the same time, it may cause problems and promote failure to keep on top of these changes.

So, as an exercise routine is quiet a large change to incorporate into your life, I would advise that you just make yourself aware of the food that you are eating and make small changes here, too, for now. Remember that a lot of small changes over time will result in a big change in the end.

I will outline some of the ideal ways to cut out bad foods and add good food choices and habits into your life:

- Cut back on, or cut out, fizzy sugary drinks – this includes energy drinks – they are no good at all.
- Cut back on chocolate, sweets and deserts. Maybe have one treat per day.
- Eat lean meat (chicken breast, lean beef and fish).
- Eat vegetables and nuts. If you snack a lot, snack on raw veggies such as carrot sticks, celery sticks and almonds instead of doughnuts, cookies and potato chips.
- Start to add more whole grains, beans, fruits, and vegetables into your diet.
- Cut down on your portion size at each meal.
- Don't cut out your favorite cheat foods altogether. Instead, eat smaller portions of this or have this only once per week.

So this is a list of things that you can work towards! But I would suggest changing one thing at a time and not making all of these changes together. If you are very strong-minded and believe that you can make all of these changes all at once and make them stick, great stuff! Do it.

CHAPTER 5

GET MOTIVATED

On the next page, I have included some motivational quotes. I have added these on whole single pages so that you can cut them out.

As I have mentioned before, I do understand how hard it can be to get motivated. I, myself, have benefitted from these motivational quotes at those times when I thought, "Hmm, it's raining outside, and I think I'll give cardio a miss today."

If these little snippets of motivation are on display in your everyday life, they can have a dramatic effect when reminding you of your goals.

I suggest cutting these out and placing them where you will always see them especially in the places you will be before your training.

Make this your priority; get these pictures pinned up before you start this routine.

Some good places to pin up one of the motivational quotes are:

- By the side of your bed.
- On top of your television set.
- As you walk into your house at eye level.
- On your fridge or snack cupboard.
- On your bathroom mirror.
- On your monitor at work or home.

Be inventive. These will only need to stay up for around 6 weeks. By then you should have cemented your routine and created a habit, and then you will no longer need them to get you motivated.

These quotes, however, will be useful for a lifetime. Don't underestimate the power of having these small pictures dotted around your life!

THINK ABOUT WHY YOU STARTED

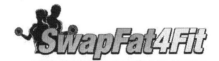

YOU DON'T HAVE TO BE GREAT TO START

BUT YOU DO HAVE TO START TO BE GREAT

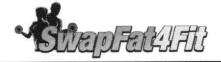

THE #1 REASON PEOPLE GIVE UP SO FAST IS THAT THEY LOOK AT HOW FAR THEY HAVE TO GO

INSTEAD OF LOOKING AT HOW FAR THEY'VE GONE ALREADY...

KEEP GOING

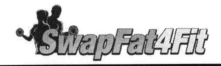

THE ONLY
BAD WORKOUT
IS THE ONE
THAT DIDN'T
HAPPEN

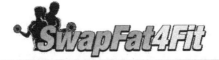

LIFE BEGINS AT THE END OF YOUR **COMFORT ZONE**

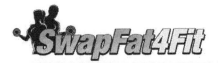

ONE HOUR OF
WORKOUT

IS 4% OF
YOUR DAY

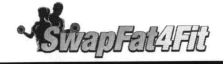

DISCIPLINE
IS THE BRIDGE
BETWEEN
GOALS AND
ACCOMPLISHMENT

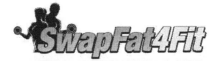

IF YOU WAIT FOR PERFECT CONDITIONS, YOU WILL NEVER **GET STARTED**

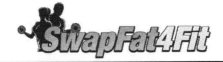

CHAPTER 6

RESISTANCE TRAINING

Over the next six weeks, we will be doing two types of exercise: *Resistance* and *Cardiovascular*. Let's take a look at *resistance training* first.

This is the part of your training where you will be targeting and working specific muscle groups in order to get them stronger and working as they should. The type of resistance training that we will be doing will build a solid foundation for your future training plans.

This part of your routine is also great for burning those extra calories, but, sadly, it is overlooked and underestimated in many occasions. So don't think that this is not helping. In fact, there are many benefits to be gained from resistance training, including boosting your fat loss.

For this routine, you should do your resistance training just after you do your cardio training, so your cardio will serve as a good warm up.

During your first six-week training routine, you will be doing 3 - 6 resistance training sessions per week.

There are a few factors that have to be considered when it comes to choosing your resistance band. You do not want to choose a band that is so tough that you can't even do the movement or you are totally exhausted after each exercise.

The point of this course is to get your muscles working, so we do not need a huge amount of resistance. You need to feel resistance and you need to be able to perform the exercise with reasonable comfort. I always say:

"It's not the size of the weight; it's how you lift it that counts."

So if you have a resistance band kit similar to the one I have suggested, you should find the resistance band that is good for you on that particular exercise. You will be able to progress through the different bands as time goes by.

If the lightest resistance band in the kit is still too tough, this is really no problem. You can just do the exercises without a band at all. If this is the case, great; you will have a lot of progression to work towards and look forward to achieving.

CHAPTER 7

CARDIO TRAINING

Cardio training is simply aerobic training, and it comes in many forms – jogging, cycling, and rowing.

This is the part of your routine where you incorporate your heart and lungs into your training routine. Cardio training is great for fat loss and the fitness of your heart and lungs, i.e. your cardio-respiratory system.

There are many ways to do cardio training. I have designed this course to be as cost-effective as possible. It is based on using walking and jogging as our cardio session choice. If you have a bicycle and would prefer to use that, you can use the same principles that I have suggested.

You can do your cardio training sessions everyday. I have outlined that you are allowed no more than one to two days off this per week for the 6-week program although these days off are not mandatory.

If you choose to drop cardio sessions, I suggest that it is planned as the same day every week. This will keep you more organized and focused.

CHAPTER 8

D.O.M.S

Delayed **O**nset **M**uscle **S**oreness. The day after you train, you may feel pain in your muscles. Let's say you first started doing body weight squats and the next day, you can feel the tops of your legs aching every time you take a step or walk up a flight of stairs. This is D.O.M.S. Although you are feeling this pain, it is important to understand that this is a very good sign! This means that you have challenged your muscles and they will develop, become stronger and help you to burn fat. If you are a total beginner you may confuse this for an injury, but the more you train, the less you will feel the effect.

It is important to be able to differentiate between D.O.M.S and an injury. A good indication of an injury will be if you feel pain in your joints or sudden muscular pain whilst you are exercising.

As this is a beginner's course, you should not have extreme D.O.M.S., and if you follow the exercise descriptions, you should not get an injury. However, if you do feel very uncomfortable performing a particular exercise because of pain. Leave that exercise out and resume training when you do not feel any pain. If the pain persists or you are unsure, please see your doctor. Remember, if you injure yourself, it may affect your progress. It is better to miss one or two exercises out than not do the training session at all.

CHAPTER 9

PREPARATION BEFORE YOU START

Before you start your six-week routine, it is a good idea to get yourself prepared. It is very important to be prepared, not just physically but mentally, too.

Make sure you have an uninterrupted 6-week period ahead of you before deciding your start date. By this, I mean don't do week 1 and 2 and then go on holiday for two weeks.

- Create your own motivational quotes or use the ones in this book and pin them up where you will always see them.
- Cut out (or keep this book handy in your training area) stages 1-6 of your workouts and pin them up somewhere, so you can tick the boxes as you finish each workout. It's best to pin these up as if they were a calendar, so you only see one week at a time – the week you are working on.
- Plan your start date. It is important to have the start date in mind before you just jump in. This will help you mentally prepare.
- Make sure you have all of the equipment that you need.
- Read through the exercises and get yourself familiar with them.
- Tell people what you are doing and when you are starting. This should give you some extra support and you may even find a training partner to do the whole thing with.

Make sure you have ticked off all of these before starting Week 1. Some of this may sound or look silly but it WILL help you out.

Week 1 – 6
Exercise Plan

CHAPTER 10

WEEK 1
"LET'S GET STARTED"

Cardio
Cardio should be done at least 5 out of 7 days per week

MON	TUES	WED	THUR	FRI	SAT	SUN

Normal walk – Find a route that is a 0.5–1 mile circuit. Don't worry about the time that this takes at first; just make sure you get into the habit of walking this route every day. Pick a landmark on this route that you believe to be around halfway.

Be aware of this landmark every time that you pass it on your sessions. We will need this later.

Time how long this walk takes you. Don't try to do it quickly, just walk and make a note of how long this takes you.

This part of the routine is working to get you fitter and burn fat. It is giving you a strong foundation and helping with one of the most important factors in any fitness routine, i.e. getting you into a routine!

It is very important that you do this circuit every training day.

Resistance

Resistance should be done 3 out of 7 days per week

MON	TUES	WED	THUR	FRI	SAT	SUN

1. Seated exercise band chest press.
   2 sets of 12 reps

2. Leg extensions with exercise band
   2 sets of 12 reps

3. Bicep curls with exercise band
   2 sets of 12 reps

4. Lateral raises with exercise band
   2 sets of 12 reps

5. Tricep kickbacks with exercise band
   2 sets of 12 reps

6. Crunches on floor, wrists to knees
   2 sets of 12 reps

7. Dorsal raises, hands on floor
   2 sets of 12 reps

CHAPTER 11

WEEK 2
"KEEP IT UP"

Cardio
Cardio should be done at least 5 out of 7 days per week.

MON	TUES	WED	THUR	FRI	SAT	SUN

Brisk walk around your route – Increase the pace, try to keep a steady pace, make a conscious effort to walk faster than you would normally. This is where the time-keeping comes in – see if you can beat your previous time. You will be surprised how much faster you can do this route. Everyday, try to beat your time without jogging. Don't worry if you don't make it or if you were faster the previous day. This is not our aim, as long as you have kept a brisk walk up all the way round, that's what we are after.

Resistance
Resistance should be done 3 out of 7 days per week

MON	TUES	WED	THUR	FRI	SAT	SUN

1. Seated exercise band chest press
   3 sets of 12 reps

2. Leg extensions with exercise band
   3 sets of 12 reps

3. Bicep curls with exercise band
   3 sets of 12 reps

4. Lateral raises with exercise band
   3 sets of 12 reps

5. Tricep kickbacks with exercise band
   3 sets of 12 reps

6. Crunches on floor, wrists to knees
   3 sets of 12 reps

7. Dorsal raises, hands on floor
   3 sets of 12 reps

CHAPTER 12

WEEK 3
"GETTING INTO ROUTINE"

Cardio
Cardio should be done at least 5 out of 7 days per week

MON	TUES	WED	THUR	FRI	SAT	SUN

Interval training – By now, you will be familiar with your route and will have been doing a brisk walk around it.

What we need to do now is to throw in a 30-second jog.

Now I have heard people say, "I have never jogged in my life."

If this is you, get that thought out of your head; it is a barrier that is holding you back, and it's going to happen. We are going to hit a slow jog for 30 seconds. (That's only half of a minute.) Once you have done this, you can carry on with your brisk walk to the end of your circuit.

Resistance
Resistance should be done 4 out of 7 days per week

MON	TUES	WED	THUR	FRI	SAT	SUN

1. Push-ups on knees
   3 sets of 12 reps

2. Swiss ball squats
   3 sets of 12 reps

3. Bicep curls with exercise band
   3 sets of 12 reps

4. Shoulder press
   3 sets of 12 reps

5. Tricep dips, feet on floor
   3 sets of 12 reps

6. Crunches on floor, hands on sides of head
   3 sets of 12 reps

7. Dorsal raises, hands on sides of head
   3 sets of 12 reps

CHAPTER 13

WEEK 4
"CEMENTING THE ROUTINE"

Cardio
Cardio should be done at least 5 out of 7 days per week

MON	TUES	WED	THUR	FRI	SAT	SUN

Start your brisk walk as normal for 2 minutes, then do a 30-second slow jog... carry on your brisk walk to your halfway point and do your second 30-second jog... carry on with your brisk walk to the end.

You will notice that this has not taken you as long as before to do your cardio.

Resistance
Resistance should be done 4 out of 7 days per week

MON	TUES	WED	THUR	FRI	SAT	SUN

1. Push-ups on knees
    3 sets of 15 reps

2. Swiss ball squats
    3 sets of 15 reps

3. Bicep curls with exercise band
    3 sets of 15 reps

4. Lateral raises with exercise band
    3 sets of 15 reps

5. Tricep kickbacks with exercise band
    3 sets of 15 reps

6. Crunches on floor, wrists to knees
    3 sets of 15 reps

7. Dorsal raises, hands on side of head
    3 sets of 15 reps

CHAPTER 14

WEEK 5
"WELL DONE! KEEP GOING"

Cardio
Cardio should be done at least 6 out of 7 days per week

MON	TUES	WED	THUR	FRI	SAT	SUN

Start your brisk walk for 5 minutes, and then for the rest of the circuit, do a 30-second jog... followed by 1 minute brisk walk... followed by another 30-second jog... followed by a brisk walk for 1 minute.

Repeat this pattern until the end of the circuit.

Resistance
Resistance should be done 4 out of 7 days per week

MON	TUES	WED	THUR	FRI	SAT	SUN

1. Full push-ups
   3 sets of 15-30 reps

2. Bodyweight squats
   3 sets of 12 reps

3. Bicep curls with exercise band
   3 sets of 12 reps

4. Shoulder press
   3 sets of 12 reps

5. Tricep dips, feet on floor
   3 sets of 12 reps

6. Swiss ball crunches
   3 sets of 12 reps

7. Bent over rows
   3 sets of 12 reps

CHAPTER 15

WEEK 6
"CONGRATULATIONS!
FIRST SIX WEEKS OF FITNESS
DOWN"

Cardio
Cardio should be done at least 6 out of 7 days per week

MON	TUES	WED	THUR	FRI	SAT	SUN

Double your circuit, doing a 30-second jog and 1-minute brisk walk all of the way round. You may notice that this takes you nearly the same amount of time to do the circuit this way as it did right at the beginning.

This cardio session will be a 2-mile course with a 30-second jog every 1 minute. It will be good enough for a sustainable fitness plan for the long-term.

If this does get too easy, you can look at reducing the brisk walk phase to 30 seconds so it becomes a 30-second jog and a 30-second brisk walk. You could also look at jogging and 30-second sprints in the future. There are many different progression options.

Resistance
Resistance should be done 4 out of 7 days per week

MON	TUES	WED	THUR	FRI	SAT	SUN

1. Full push-ups
    3 sets of 15-50 reps

2. Bodyweight squats
    3 sets of 25-50 reps

3. Bicep curls with exercise band
    3 sets of 25-50 reps

4. Shoulder press
    3 sets of 25-50 reps

5. Tricep dips, feet on floor
    3 sets of 25-50 reps

6. Swiss ball crunches
    3 sets of 25-50 reps

7. Bent over rows
    3 sets of 25-50 reps.

WHAT DO YOU THINK SO FAR?

I am always eager to hear what you think of my exercise routines.

I would really appreciate it if you left a review and rating on the online retail store from which you made this purchase and tell others about your experience.

Please take a few moments to do this if you have enjoyed this book so far.

Thanks for the feedback! ☺

Exercise
Descriptions

EXERCISE DESCRIPTIONS

SEATED CHEST PRESS

Start/Finish Position   Top Of Movement

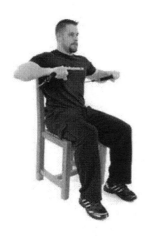 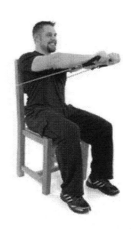

Target muscle group is shown below:

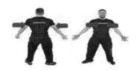

DESCRIPTION OF EXERCISE
(SEATED CHEST PRESS)

Attach stirrups to each end of the band, cross the band around a high-backed chair (See 'More Information' section).

Start position:
Sit on the chair with the band attached, ensuring that your back is straight, your feet are flat to the floor and you are looking straight in front of you. Hold the stirrups in each hand with palms facing the floor ensuring that your forearms are parallel to the floor. Your hands should be in line with your chest and you should feel a slight resistance from the band.

Movement:
Keeping your forearms parallel to the floor, straighten your arms out in front of you and bring your hands to meet each other at the end of the movement so they touch when your arms are fully extended. You should also exhale as you do this. Return to the start position whilst breathing in and you have completed one rep.

You should feel this in your chest.

LEG EXTENSION

Start/Finish Position.. Top Of Movement

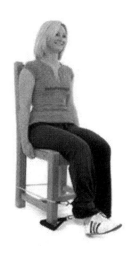 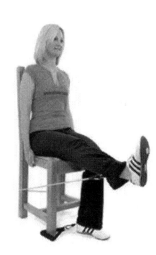

Target muscle group is shown below:

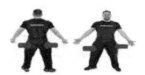

DESCRIPTION OF EXERCISE
(LEG EXTENSION)

Attach the ankle straps to both ends of the band (See 'More Information' section).

Start Position:
Sit on a chair or bench, place one end of the resistance band either under your left foot or wrapped around the rear right chair leg.
Attach the ankle strap around your right ankle. If you do not have one of these, you can make a loop in the band. Grasp sides of chair with your hands for support. Keep the toes on the foot of your working leg pointed up.

Movement:
As you exhale, extend your right leg to the point just before you lock out and try to get your lower leg parallel to the floor. From this point, keeping your leg straight, lift your upper leg towards the ceiling.
Return to the start position by bending your knee whilst breathing in. This completes one rep.

Finish your set and swap legs.

BICEP CURL

Start/Finish Position   Top Of Movement

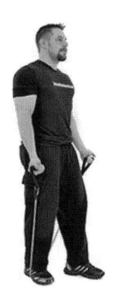 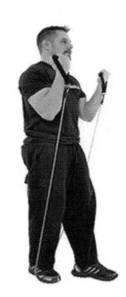

Target muscle group is shown below:

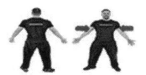

DESCRIPTION OF EXERCISE
(BICEP CURL)

Attach stirrups to each end of the band.

Start position:
Hold a stirrup in each hand, step forward with one foot securing the middle of the band under the rear foot. Keep your palms facing forward and allow your arms to fall naturally at your sides with elbows slightly bent, eyes looking straight and your back flat.

Movement:
Whilst breathing out, bring your forearms up to as parallel with your upper arm as possible and squeezing your bicep.
You should not rotate your palms inwards, your palms should be facing the front of your shoulder at the top of this movement (maximum contraction). Breathe in as you return to the starting position. This completes one rep.

You should feel this in your biceps, the front of your upper arm.

LATERAL RAISES

Start/Finish Position   Top Of Movement

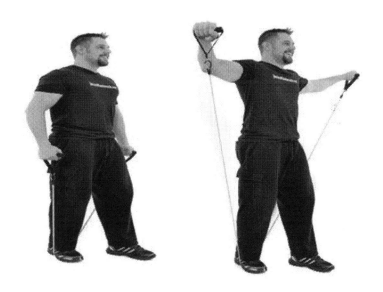

Target muscle group is shown below:

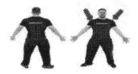

DESCRIPTION OF EXERCISE
(LATERAL RAISES)

Attach stirrups to each end of the band.

Start position:
Hold a stirrup in each hand, step forward with one foot securing the middle of the band under the rear foot. Keep your palms facing inwards, your elbows slightly bent and locked, eyes looking straight and your back flat.

Movement:
Whilst breathing out and keeping your elbows and wrists locked, bring your arms parallel or just above parallel to the floor. Breathe in on returning to the start position. This completes one rep.

You should feel this in your shoulders.

TRICEP KICKBACKS

Start/Finish Position   Top Of Movement

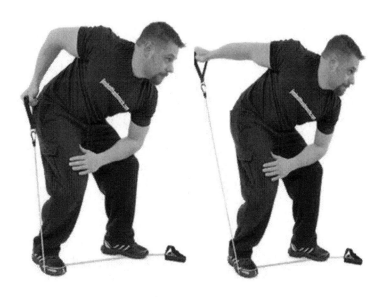

Target muscle group is shown below:

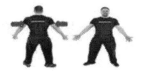

DESCRIPTION OF EXERCISE
(TRICEP KICKBACKS)

Attach stirrups to each end of the band.

Start position:
Place the exercise band on the floor and step on it around 12" from the stirrup attachment with your right foot – this will be your front foot. (This will vary from person to person. You are looking to have tension on the band at the starting position). Bring your left foot behind you to give yourself a good platform.

Keeping your knees bent and your feet where they are, bend over to pick the stirrup up with your right hand. Stay bent over with a flat back and pull your upper arm to your side and keep your elbow in. You should by now feel the tension from the band. If you don't, bring your right foot closer to the stirrup. Twist your palm so it is facing behind you.

Movement:
Keeping your upper arm parallel with the floor and your palm facing backwards whilst breathing out, move your lower arm towards the sky to the point just before it locks out. Then bring this back to the starting position as you breathe in. This completes one rep.

Once the set is done, switch arms. Do the same thing again with your left foot leading.

CRUNCHES
(WRISTS TO KNEES)

Start/Finish Position   Top Of Movement

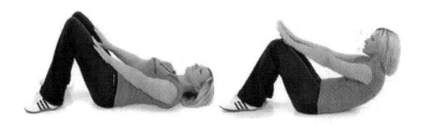

Target muscle group is shown below:

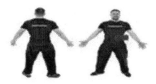

DESCRIPTION OF EXERCISE
(CRUNCHES, WRISTS TO KNEES)

Start position:
Lay flat on your back and bring your knees up so that your feet are flat on the floor about shoulder width apart. Place the tips of your fingers on the side of your head.
DO NOT CLASP YOUR HANDS BEHIND YOUR HEAD.

Movement:
As you breathe out, slowly lift your upper body off the floor whilst sliding your palms towards your knees. You should aim to get your wrists to your knees. Once at the top of this movement, breathe in and lower your upper body back to the start position. This completes one rep.

DORSAL RAISES
(HANDS ON FLOOR)

Start/Finish Position   Top Of Movement

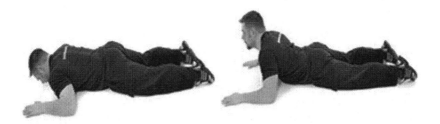

Target muscle group is shown below:

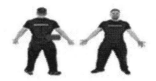

DESCRIPTION OF EXERCISE
(DORSAL, RAISES HANDS ON FLOOR)

Start position:
Lay face down on the floor, pointing your toes so the tops of your feet are also in contact with the floor. Your lower arms should be in contact with the floor and at right angles to your upper arm with palms facing down.

Movement:
As you breathe out, bring your upper body off the floor assisting slightly with your hands. Once at the top of the movement, lower your upper body in the same way whilst breathing in. This completes one rep.

(It is important to remember that this is a small range of movement so don't strain yourself too much at the top of the movement.)

PUSH-UPS ON KNEES

Start/Finish Position   Top Of Movement

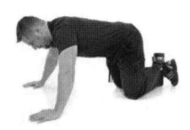 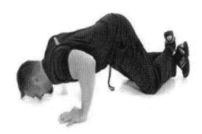

Target muscle group is shown below:

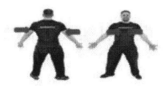

DESCRIPTION OF EXERCISE
(PUSH-UPS ON KNEES)

Start position:
Get to a position on the floor so you are on your hands and knees. Your hands should be about shoulder width apart and in line with your face.

Movement:
Keep your back straight and lower your upper body towards the floor by bending your elbows and breathing in.
Once you're at the bottom of this movement, whilst breathing out, raise your upper body back to the starting position. This completes one rep.

If you can do more than 30, move to full push-ups.

SWISS BALL SQUATS

Start/Finish Position   Top Of Movement

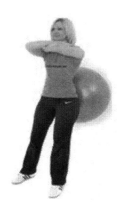 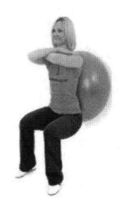

Target muscle group is shown below:

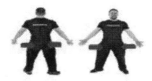

DESCRIPTION OF EXERCISE
(SWISS BALL SQUATS)

Start position:
Stand with your back against a flat wall, then position the ball in between your back and the wall so it rests in your lower back.
Keep your feet hip-width apart, slightly in front of your shoulders.

Movement:
As you breathe in, bend your knees until your quads (Upper legs) are parallel to the ground. (The exercise ball will roll and end up between your shoulder blades).
Then push back through your heels to the starting position whilst breathing out.

Ensure that you are always looking straight ahead or slightly up. This will help you keep good posture. This completes one rep.

SHOULDER PRESS

Start/Finish Position   Top Of Movement

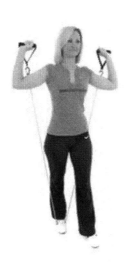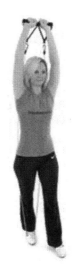

Target muscle group is shown below:

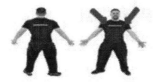

note; please skip this exercise or check with your doctor if you have a known heart condition.

DESCRIPTION OF EXERCISE
(SHOULDER PRESS)

Attach stirrups to each end of the band.

Start position:
Hold a stirrup in each hand, step forward with one foot securing the middle of the band under the rear foot. Keep your palms facing forward and in line with your chin. Your eyes should be looking straight and your back should be flat.

Movement:
Whilst breathing out and maintaining your posture, push the stirrups above your head as high as you can, bringing the two stirrups together to touch at the top of the movement. You should not let your elbows lock. As you breathe in, lower your arms back to the starting position. This completes one rep.

TRICEP DIPS
(FEET ON FLOOR)

Start/Finish Position Top Of Movement

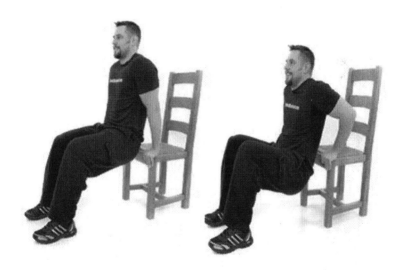

Target muscle group is shown below:

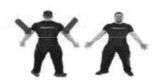

DESCRIPTION OF EXERCISE
(TRICEP DIPS, FEET ON FLOOR)

Start position:
Sit with your back to a bench or chair and place your hands so that your fingers are pointing forward and taking your body weight.
You should now be in a seated position with your feet flat on the floor.

Movement:
As you breathe in, lower your body, allowing your elbows to flare out naturally to the side as you lower your body towards the floor. You should lower yourself only to the point that you feel the stretch on your triceps (upper rear arms). Once at the bottom of the movement, raise your body back up to the starting position as you breathe out. This completes one rep.

CRUNCHES
(HANDS ON SIDES OF HEAD)

Start/Finish Position   Top Of Movement

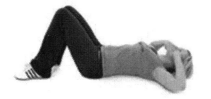 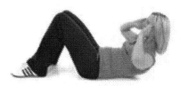

Target muscle group is shown below:

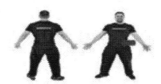

DESCRIPTION OF EXERCISE
(CRUNCHES, HANDS ON SIDES OF HEAD)

Start position:
Lay flat on your back and bring your knees up so your feet are flat on the floor about shoulder width apart.

Movement:
As you breathe out, slowly lift your upper body off the floor whilst sliding your palms towards your knees. You should aim to get your wrists to your knees.

Once at the top of this movement, breathe in and lower your upper body back to the start position. This completes one rep.

FULL PUSH-UPS

Start/Finish Position   Top Of Movement

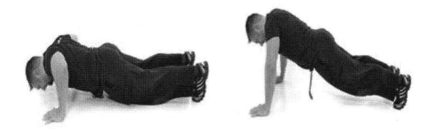

Target muscle group is shown below:

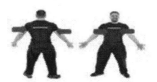

DESCRIPTION OF EXERCISE
(FULL PUSHUPS)

Start position:
Get into a position on the floor so your hands are about shoulder width apart and in line with your mid/upper chest. You should keep your back flat and take the weight of your body. Make sure that you do not dip your head.

Movement:
Keep your back straight and lower your upper body towards the floor by bending your elbows whilst breathing in. Once you are at the bottom of this movement, as you breathe out, raise your upper body back to the starting position. This completes one rep.

BODYWEIGHT SQUATS

Start/Finish Position   Top Of Movement

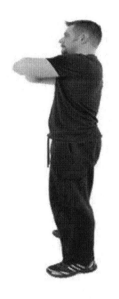 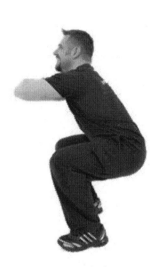

Target muscle group is shown below:

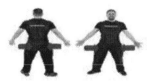

DESCRIPTION OF EXERCISE
(BODYWEIGHT SQUATS)

Start position:

Stand with your feet hip-width apart, toes slightly turned out and your arms across your chest. Focus on a point on a wall or in the distances that is eye level or higher and look at this throughout the movement. This will help you keep your posture and maintain correct form.

Movement:

Keeping your feet flat on the floor, as you breathe in, bend your knees until your quads (Upper legs) are parallel to the ground. Push back through your heels to the starting position. Whilst breathing out. Ensure that you are always looking straight ahead or slightly up. This will help you keep good posture. This completes one rep.

TRICEP DIPS
(HEELS ON FLOOR)

Start/Finish Position Top Of Movement

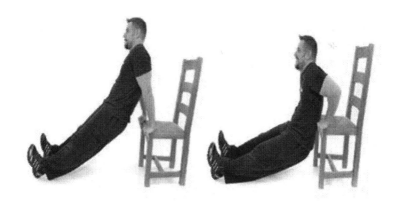

Target muscle group is shown below:

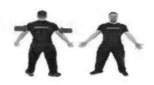

DESCRIPTION OF EXERCISE
(TRICEP DIPS, HEELS ON FLOOR)

For this exercise, I would make sure the chair or bench is against a wall so it does not slip.

Start position:
Sit with your back to a bench or chair and place your hands so that your fingers are pointing forward and taking your bodyweight.
You should now be in a seated position with your feet flat on the floor. Stay in this position but straighten your legs out in front of you so that your heels are on the floor and toes are pointed up.

Movement:
As you breathe in, lower your body, allowing your elbows to flare out naturally to the side as you lower your body towards the floor.
You should lower yourself only to the point that you feel the stretch on your triceps (upper rear arms). Once at the bottom of the movement, raise your body back up to the starting position as you breathe out. This completes one rep.

SWISS BALL CRUNCHES

Start/Finish Position   Top Of Movement

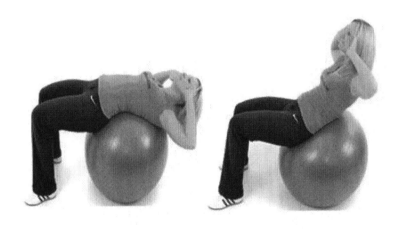

Target muscle group is shown below:

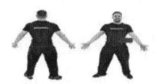

DESCRIPTION OF EXERCISE
(SWISS BALL CRUNCHES)

Start position:
Sit on the swiss-ball with your feet flat on the ground. Walk your feet forward so the swiss-ball rolls up your back and you are in a lying position. The swiss-ball should be in your mid to lower back and you should be looking up at the sky.
Place your fingertips on the side of your head.
DO NOT CLASP YOUR HANDS BEHIND YOUR HEAD.

Movement:
Keeping your feet flat on the floor, you should lift your shoulder blades up. This will put immediate tension on your abdominals. You should breathe out as you do this.
Your lower back should not lose contact with the swiss-ball and your eyes should be in line with the sky at a 45-degree angle. Once you reach the top of the movement, lower your shoulders to the starting position whilst breathing in. This completes one rep.

BENT OVER ROWS

Start/Finish Position Top Of Movement

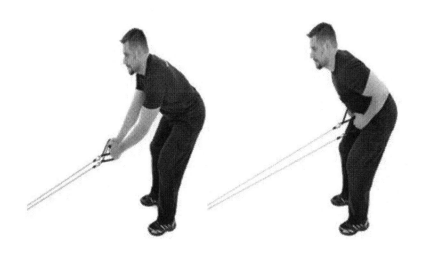

Target muscle group is shown below:

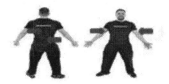

DESCRIPTION OF EXERCISE
(BENT OVER ROWS)

Attach the stirrups to both ends of the band, loop through the door attachment (See 'More Information' section).

Start position:
Stand with your feet shoulder width apart, bend over so your upper body is just above parallel to the floor and your back is straight. Take up the slack of the resistance band so that you have tension when your hands are in front of your body as illustrated.
Keep your head up and look forward at all times.

Movement:
As you breathe out, pull the bands into your body, I always aim for my belly button *(When you row, stay low)*. Once at the top of the movement, return to the start position as you inhale. This completes one rep.

Remember to keep your head up, chest out and back flat throughout the movement.

More
Information

CHEST PRESS

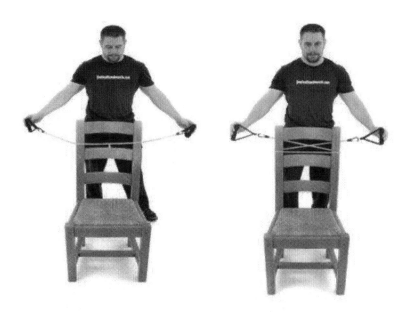

DESCRIPTION

Attach the stirrups to both ends of the band.

Position 1: Loop the band around the back of the chair.
Position 2: Cross the exercise band over at the back of the chair.

LEG EXTENSIONS

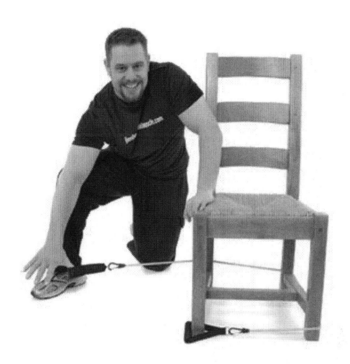

DESCRIPTION

Attach a stirrup to one end of the band and an ankle strap to the other.

Position 1: Place the stirrup through the front chair leg.
Position 2: Pass the exercise band around the opposite front leg and continue to wrap around the rear chair legs until the ankle strap meets the front stirrup.
(Note that this example shows the set up for right leg training only)

BENT OVER ROWS

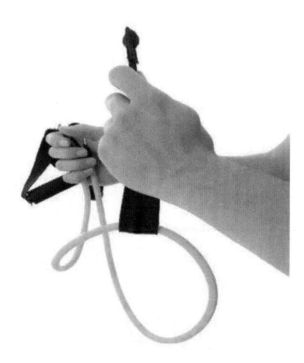

DESCRIPTION

Attach the stirrups to both ends of the band, loop through the door attachment.

Before you start the exercise, ensure that you have even lengths of exercise band on each side of the door attachment.
This shows the door attachment that came with my exercise band kit. Different kits will have varying attachments.
When using these attachments, ensure that you are using against a closed door that opens outwards to your working position. This will give extra stability.

WHERE DO YOU GO FROM HERE?

Now that you have introduced a home workout routine into your life and, hopefully, established a good set of habits that will enable you to develop the body and weight goals of your dreams, you do not have to sit back on your laurels; you can step it up a gear and get your results even quicker!

I have written a follow-up to this book that will push your fitness to the next level. This can also be done from the comfort of your own home.

I have designed the next six-week routine to run as a nice challenging progression to the routine outlined in this book.

The next book in this series is called:

"Home Workout Circuit Training"

The routines from "Home Workout Circuit Training" use a fusion of cardio and resistance training to demonstrate a whole new way of utilizing some of the movements already learned in this book.

Training in this way can massively boost your muscle strength and tone and also make a huge difference in your fat burning goals!

Check it out and remember that I am always more than happy to answer any questions that you may have.

Good luck!

ONE LAST THING

I would like to take this opportunity to send you a sincere "thank you" for purchasing this book. It really means a lot to me that you chose this over all of the other competition.

I would also like to let you know that this was self-published. This means that I have had no help with promotion or financial backing in the writing, editing, design and publishing process of this book.

I strongly believe that this is a very good guide and I would like to get it into the hands of as many people in need of real weight loss and fitness help as possible.

Therefore, I would be delighted if you would mention this to your friends if you think that they will benefit from it. Facebook it, tweet it, blog it! ☺

There is also a mission statement on the swapfat4fit.com website. I truly love to hear when someone has gained results from reading my work.

It would be great if you could swing by here, give it a read and leave a comment on the page.

Many thanks, good luck and I look forward to hearing from you!

All the very best,
Jim.

ALSO BY JAMES ATKINSON

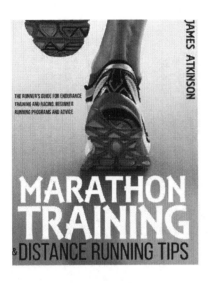

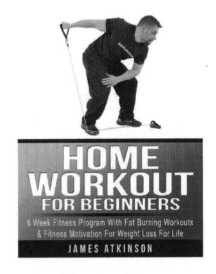

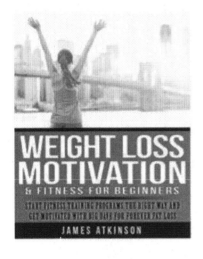

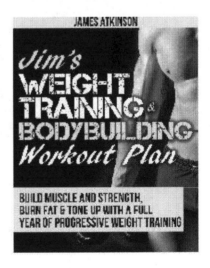

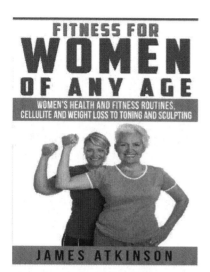

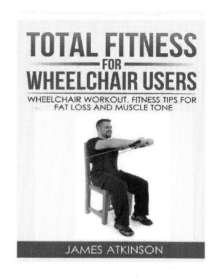

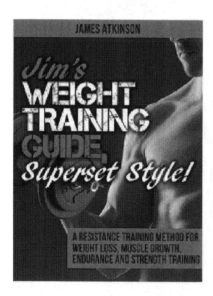

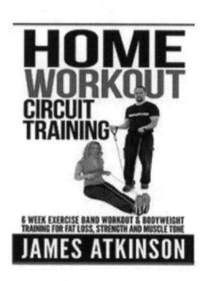

CONNECT WITH JIM

Visit Jim's blog for more great advice on diet, training, healthy recipes, motivation and more: www.jimshealthandmuscle.com

Get regular updates on Facebook when you "like" and "follow" Jim's pages here:

Facebook.com/JimsHealthandMuscle
Facebook.com/SwapFat4Fit

Catch the trends. Follow Jim on Twitter here:

@JimsHM

Made in the USA
San Bernardino, CA
28 January 2018